I0091434

THE PREPARED PATIENT

For my incredibly strong, courageous and
beautiful mother and aunt who, along with
millions of others have suffered unnecessarily due
to errors, miscommunications and misinformation

For the families who grieve the loss or suffering
of a loved one due to medical errors or hospital
acquired infections

For the many doctors, nurses and healthcare
professionals who rise each day with the sole
intent of helping others

THE PREPARED PATIENT

Simple Tools That May
Save Your Life

Christine M. Gannon, CEO, M.Ed.

Copyright © 2020 Christine M. Gannon

The Prepared Patient

Simple Tools That May Save Your Life

Christine M. Gannon, CEO, M.Ed.

978-0-578-76926-4

All rights reserved. This book is protected under the copyright
laws of the United States of America. This book may not be
copied or reprinted for commercial gain or profit.

For worldwide distribution. Printed in the U.S.A.

CONTENTS

INTRODUCTION

The monitor slowed to a complete and hard stop leaving behind and a loud, piercing noise, complimented by a green flat line. Her heart had finally given out. Even though her organs had shut down hours before, her heart had been the only thing still going. For many nights after my mother's passing in a local hospital, I was haunted by the fact that I was far from equipped to have dealt with the situation. I was a corporate executive, not a doctor or a nurse.

I was asked to make decisions that I was not educated to make, nor was I in any emotional or physical state to adequately make such decisions. I felt hopeless, helpless and regretful that I wasn't prepared to quickly respond and react in a way that may have prevented the medical errors that ensued. I was also confused by the absence of education at the hospital or from a doctor's office or healthcare agency during this time. Didn't that always happen? Wasn't someone there to explain things in detail and provide an in-depth review of options, risks and recommendations? Whose responsibility was it to navigate a complex healthcare situation? Mine and rightfully so as the responsible party for her given her incapacity.

Reflecting back over the situation, I was convinced there had to be a way to become pro-active so that if I found myself in a similar situation for myself or a loved one, I would have a better understanding of what to do and feel equipped with critical information to support the challenges that lie ahead.

This realization launched the passion behind the mission of Just for Patients, a 501c3 established to educate, raise awareness and provide resources for patient navigation and advocacy.

In the beginning of this journey, on almost a daily basis I thought to myself, "If I have experienced this, others must have too." I began my research to find out who was helping these "others" that found themselves in medical situations without the proper education, tools and knowledge. It couldn't just be doctors, nurses and healthcare professionals. During one of my many late-night research marathons online, I came across a wonderful organization, Bedside Advocates™ in Boston, Massachusetts originally started by the esteemed and late Dr. Jonathan Fine. I eagerly engaged him in conversation via email and phone calls and subsequently took a trip to Boston where he provided invaluable mentorship, encouragement and shared in the vision of my mission, which was his as well. He became a dear friend and mentor to whom I am deeply indebted.

This book serves as a tool and a starting point for every mother, father, sister, brother, daughter, son, cousin, aunt, uncle or friend who would like to be more in control of decisions made about their healthcare or those they love. This is a tool to help doctors help you! This is a means to become an active participant in your healthcare – even if only to ask the right questions to ensure the right procedures are being done.

This is a way for you to insure you have the right information available for a routine doctor's appointment or a hospital stay. This book will be the first step to equip you to navigate and advocate for yourself or a loved one and get the information you need to make important healthcare decisions.

My hope is that you read this and act! May you be motivated to track your prescriptions, your lab work, surgeries, tests and anything that relates to the wellbeing of your body, mind and spirit. Be informed and advocate for yourself and loved ones! But most importantly,

...be blessed in health!

"Take care of your body. It's the only place you have to live."

Jim Rohn

How to Use This Book

- Read this book once before you begin to gather records, information and files. Take time to deeply understand the compelling reasons and YOUR why as to the importance and the benefit of being a critical player in healthcare decisions that are presented for you or a loved one.

- After you have read this book, determine where it would be easiest for you to start. Remember this is for you, a loved one or friend. This applies across the board. It might be that you take time to clearly outline prescriptions and supplements. Depending on the situation, this could be a quick effort and take minimal time **or** it may require you to spend devoted time listing each medication or supplement, dosage amount and frequency. Either way, this book is a process and a journey that requires no pressure to complete ASAP. You'll find the necessary tools and resources to help you accomplish this in the Appendix and on our website, www.justforpatients.org.

- After tackling the easiest step first, eagerly begin the next section. If you feel overwhelmed, enlist the help of a good friend to help you or just listen to your feelings and offer support.

- Remember, this isn't a race. There isn't a timeline or deadline for completion. Take it at your own pace and one step or section at a time. Before you know its complete and only requires minimal updates as you have changes to your healthcare. You'll be prepared. Preparation often brings peace of mind.

- Share the information with doctor's and caregiver's and loved ones. Keep a copy online or in a place where you keep important documents. This is a critical step in the process to taking more control over your or a loved one's healthcare. Set dates on your calendar to maintain your information so that it remains current. This is especially important if you have more than one doctor or specialist.

- Take time to celebrate when you are finished! You have just completed taking a step to actively participating in your healthcare and potentially avoiding a medical error for yourself or a loved one.

- These documents could be organized by health issue making it even easier to address multiple health challenges, when needed. It also can provide a helpful way to address questions for specific issues with specialists.

"The best preparation for tomorrow is doing your best today."

H. Jackson Brown Jr., P.S. I Love You

CHAPTER 1

Reality Check

ROSEMARY'S STORY

Had I known then what I know today, the numerous medical errors that plagued my mother's healthcare experience may have been avoided. Her care, albeit in a well-established and well-regarded, award winning hospital, ultimately led to her death and weeks of suffering.

Entering the ER with shortness of breath and an asthma attack, it never occurred to me that a few hours later, she would be supported by breathing tube and placed in ICU under constant surveillance due to a nurse forgetting she had left her alone in the restroom. Why had I left her alone so late at night? Why had I trusted a stranger, although a trained profession, to ensure my mother would be safe and secure thru the night, when the staff on call had so many other patients *and emergencies to attend to? Questions like these and many more kept me awake at night for years.*

Today, we find ourselves seeking the best healthcare possible in a very complex system. Doctors, nurses and healthcare professionals find themselves in the very same situation. We are all a part of this system, trying to either obtain care or deliver care. Regardless, neither has the better position.

MEDICAL ERRORS: HOW DO THEY HAPPEN?

A recent Johns Hopkins study claims more than 250,000 people in the U.S. die every year from medical errors. Other reports claim the numbers to be as high as 440,000, making it the 3rd leading cause of death in the United States.[1] With these staggering statistics, which doesn't account for the errors and deaths that are not reported as an error, it is imperative to be prepared for your healthcare experiences as much as possible.

Having critical healthcare information in an easy to access and easy to read format may mitigate and save lives in some situations. Being an advocate for yourself or having one participating for you, to be able to ask critical questions and share valuable information is a critical way to prevent misunderstanding, duplication of testing, confusion and potentially a medical error.

Dr. Martin Makary of the Johns Hopkins University School of Medicine defines a death due to medical error "as one that is caused by inadequately skilled staff, error in judgment or care, a system defect or a preventable adverse effect. This includes computer breakdowns, mix-ups with the doses or types of medications administered to patients and surgical complications that go undiagnosed."[2] Let's take a closer look.

The US alone will need to hire 2.3 million new health care workers by 2025 in order to adequately take care of its aging population, a new report finds.[3] Dr. Jason Narlock, senior consultant with Mercer says "When there are fewer nurses available to handle a bigger volume of patients, it **adversely affects patient outcomes because of nursing burnout**," said Narlock. "Patients are more likely to be readmitted after 30 days of first being seen. They can also be at a higher risk of a hospital acquired infection. When patients are readmitted, it puts more pressure on physicians who are already handling a heavy patient load."[4]

Inadequate and/or poor communication has been a leading factor in approximately 1,744 patient deaths with over $1.7 billion in malpractice costs in the United States in the past five years, according to a study published in FierceHealthcare.[5] "In a retrospective review of 14,000 in-hospital deaths, communication errors were found to be the lead cause, twice as frequent as errors due to inadequate clinical skill," notes a 2006 study in the Clinical Biochemist Review.[6] Communication is a relatively easy fix and because it means that patient deaths are preventable with process improvement in the communications sector of a hospital or doctor's office, it should be considered a priority to ensure communication channels are clear.

LACK OF ADEQUATE NUMBERS OF NURSING STAFF CAN IMPACT PATIENT WELL-BEING IN A NUMBER OF WAYS

HIGHER PATIENT MORTALITY

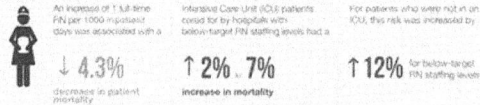

↓ 4.3%   ↑ 2% - 7%   ↑ 12%

MORE MEDICATION ERRORS

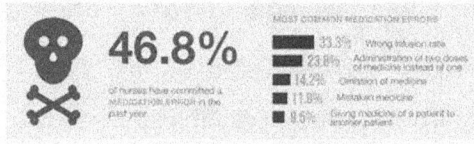

46.8%

Source: Bradley University's Online MSN-FNP program

This is where your responsibility for communication becomes critical. Keeping the lines of communication open between you, your loved one and healthcare professionals treating the patient, could become the difference between life and death. Documenting what's happening at doctor's visits, tele-health video/calls, hospital stay's, ER visits, conversations, testing, and prescriptions can be a life-saving element of your healthcare experience. As the patient or caregiver, you can only control so much. Ensuring that your communication is clear, current and accurate is significant and within your control.

"What is left unsaid in the exam room is not necessarily forgotten by the patient. Research found

21

that 9% of patients had something they wanted to ask their physicians but did not. Subsequently, they reported less improvement in their symptoms."[7]

SEVEN MINUTES

With the average doctor's visit lasting approximately seven minutes or less, your ability to have critical information available and ready to review is key to participating in your healthcare decisions. While doctor's offices have records, they maintain, have you read these files, online or in a file folder? Most often they are incomplete or do not fully outline your healthcare issues. If there are multiple conditions involved, most often these interdependencies are not noted or included in diagnosis or records. In many cases, doctors don't call multiple providers or understand the issues that you are seeing another healthcare provider for. With countless patients to see, doctors quickly assess and prescribe, in hopes of quickly healing your current ailment or issue and restoring health.

With the exception of a pandemic (COVID-19) or unprecedented healthcare crisis, our healthcare system is continually undergoing a transformation and is works hard to become more reliable, safe, patient friendly and provide healthcare professionals the time needed to adequately serve the community they practice in. Even with constant process improvements to the system, it is up to you and I to ensure we provide critical information, ask probing questions and follow up where there is confusion or lack of information in each healthcare situation we find ourselves or a loved one in. The following chapters help you begin this journey with a clearer understanding of how to be prepared, feel empowered and participate more fully in the healthcare you receive.

> *"It is health that is real wealth and not pieces of gold and silver."*
> **Mahatma Gandhi**

We are all part of this system as it is today. Those who care for you also get ill and experience the same challenges as everyone else. But, with all its imperfections, this industry has made great advances in healthcare and most of us will have a better quality of life because of it.

"An ounce of prevention is worth a pound of cure."

Benjamin Franklin

CHAPTER 2

HealthCare Reform and You

ROSEMARY'S STORY

. . . So many doctors, so many opinions and no history readily available to share with the hospital staff. In the early days of her hospital stay, I was completely unprepared for the amount of information I needed to have with me to assist any nurse, doctor or intern with recommendations for my mother. One nurse insisted she needed insulin for her diabetes. Another insisted she needed chemotherapy for her cancer, neither of which were the current diagnosis. By the grace of God, she'd never had cancer nor diabetes. While I was astounded and frightened, I soon realized that having a clear understanding of all aspects of her health situation was critically necessary to me as the family member in charge. Actively participating every moment, asking questions regardless of how ignorant

they may have sounded, and ensuring the medication given was for her and not the patient in the next bed, was crucial to her survival.

In early 2010, the journey toward healthcare reform reached a historic milestone with legislation that extended health care coverage to all Americans and imposed restrictions on the insurance industry. The changes, initiated in 2014, have been recently updated in light of the incoming Trump Administration. Some of the key provisions of the Affordable Care Act (ACA) of 2014[8] were:

- Beginning in 2014, any individual who didn't obtain insurance coverage would pay a penalty of $95 or 1% of their income, whichever is greater. That penalty rose to $695 or 2.5% of their income in 2016.

Update: The 2017 tax overhaul legislation reduced the penalty for not having insurance to $0.

- Medicaid expansion was a key part of the 2014 ACA. The federal government helped pay for states that chose to expand Medicaid eligibility beyond families to include all low-income adults, and to raise the income threshold, so that more people would be eligible. So far, 37 states and Washington have opted to expand Medicaid.

Update: Under the Trump administration, with approval from the federal government, states can now require Medicaid beneficiaries to prove with documentation that they either work or go to school. "When you consider that, less than five years ago, Medicaid was expanded to nearly 15 million new working-age adults, it's fair that states want to add community engagement requirements for those with the ability to meet them. It's easier to give someone a card; it's much harder to build a ladder to help people climb their way out of poverty. But even though it is harder, it's the right thing to do."[9]

- Payments from the federal government to insurance companies to motivate them to stay in the ACA insurance exchanges and help keep premiums down.

Update: The Trump administration stopped paying subsidies to insurers in 2017. Employers with 50 or more workers face fines for not providing insurance coverage. Businesses with smaller workforces, though, will be exempt. Companies will receive tax credits to help buy insurance if they have 25 or fewer employees and a workforce with an average wage of up to $50,000.[10]

- The ACA initially established rules that health plans sold on HealthCare.gov and state exchanges had to cover people with preexisting conditions and had to provide certain "essential benefits." This limited any short-term insurance policies that did not provide those benefits to a maximum duration of three months.[11]

Update: The Trump administration issued a rule last year that allowed these short-term plans to last 364 days and to be renewable for three years.

- The Right to Try Act effective May of 2018 (new) lets people living with terminal diseases try experimental drugs that have passed through early-stage clinical trials and have not secured approval from the Food and Drug

Administration for use by the general public. The idea is to give people who have exhausted all other treatment options access to potentially life-saving- or -prolonging drugs.[12]

- Hospital price transparency, effective January of [13]2019 (new) requires all hospital to annually post an updated list of the charges for all of their services, known as a chargemaster.[14]

- President Trump has pledged to curb the opioid crisis. The October 2018 bill he signed included measures to increase access to addiction treatment, open more opioid recovery centers and reduce opiate prescriptions. The legislation received bipartisan support.[15]

- As of March 2020, "Insurance providers can cover COVID-19 treatment and testing for patients with Affordable Care Act catastrophic plans before the deductible is met and without requiring cost-sharing."[16]

- The CMS' Center for Medicare & Medicaid Innovation will test a program for Medicare

Part D enhanced plans that will cap out-of-pocket costs for insulin at $35 a month.

The Part D Senior Savings Model could potentially save beneficiaries in participating plans an average of $446 per year. The savings would apply to a broad set of formulary insulins, including rapid-acting, short-acting, intermediate-acting, and long-acting insulins. The goal of the Part D Senior Savings Model is to enable consistent, predictable access to medications to help improve the total cost of care for those with diabetes. The department predicts that the program could save the government more than $250 million during a five-year period, in large part due to drug companies paying additional discounts. The pilot program will begin January 1, 2021, with participating insurers.

For the latest information related to the Health Care Reform Act, login to https://www.hhs.gov/.

With all this new information, it's critically important for you to understand how your coverage is affected before you or your loved one encounter an issue or need a test. Take time to review your medical insurance as appropriate and ensure the coverage you have; is the coverage you need. "Make sure you understand your plan. Keep those benefits documents you get when you sign up for your insurance plan handy. They can provide great info on what you'll pay for different types of services, and what the rules of your insurance plan are—like whether you need to choose an in-network primary care physician or if you need referrals to see a specialist. Following the rules will help you ensure that you get quality care at a significant savings."[17]

Have someone help with understanding your healthcare plans and/or bills if they are confusing. "If you receive a large bill for services—following an ER visit or surgery, for example—and you don't understand how to read it, hire a medical billing advocate to assist you," suggests Ruth Linden, founder of Tree of Life Advocates (treeoflifehealthadvocates. com) in San Francisco. "They will not charge you if everything is in order. On the other hand, if errors or a questionable charge is found, the typical billing advocate may charge you one-third to one-half of the amount they save you. Your cost savings could run into thousands of dollars." This can be especially important if you're dealing with a complex medical issue that requires significant—and expensive—care. Some insurance companies have even begun offering their own advocates, such as UnitedHealthcare's Advocate4Me program, which provides a single point of contact with an expert who can help you understand your coverage and find the help you need.[18]

Whether it's health care reform, understanding your healthcare plan and/or benefits, it is important to know what you have available to you, in the current situation you are in. Research online and/or enlist the help of a navigator/advocate to guide you and help you uncover key information that will make life easier.

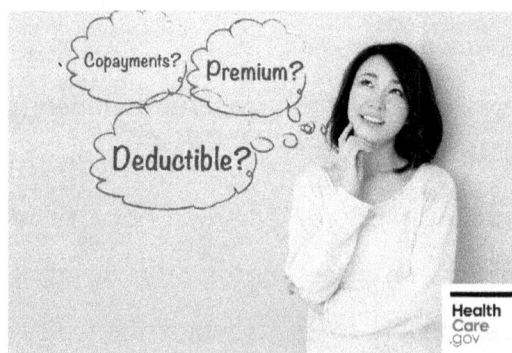

CHAPTER 3

The Prepared Patient Prescription ™

ROSEMARY'S STORY

. . . 'You're on hospital time now,' the nurse explained as I got increasingly frustrated with the lack of urgency and movement to obtain a feeding tube for my mother who had not had any nourishment for 7 days. 'Most of our patients can sustain 10 days without the feeding tube' she recanted. I had to continually remind myself that these professionals were here to help, not intentionally hurt. However, I put a call into the doctor to ask if there was any way we could expedite the process – was there a way to insert a feeding tube and see if she was able to recover from the prior medical events of the last couple days. With his help and 24 hours later, a feeding tube was placed and the 'liquid gold' as we called it, began to drip slowly into her body. As expected, she began to

show improvement in her vital signs and her body had nourishment to continue healing.

The Prepared Patient Prescription™ is an outline of simple steps to help you take more control of the healthcare received for you or your loved ones and experience healthcare in a more transparent way.

By following these simple steps, you have the opportunity to gain peace of mind that you have put in motion the right actions to help you advocate for the right level of engagement from your doctor or other healthcare professional. This also provides a tool to create a partnership, increased communication and better knowledge of the healthcare you or a loved one are receiving and why. This protocol can work whether remote (during a pandemic like COVID-19) or in a typical in-personal appointment, emergency or follow up visit.

The Prepared Patient Prescription™

STEP ONE: *ACKNOWLEDGE HEALTHCARE PROFESSIONALS ARE IN THE BUSINESS TO HELP*

One of first steps in becoming an active participant in your healthcare is to ensure your mindset is one that acknowledges healthcare professionals. They may be showing up for day one of a (3) day 12-hour shift sequence energized and ready to go or they may be a professional who is tired, stressed, overworked and potentially close to burn out. Whatever the case, they are in the business to help. Most, if not all, are truly doing the absolute best job they can, given the situation. As a reminder, healthcare professional call it a "practice" and there is a reason for that. They are practicing and using the best information they have with their experience, education and collective wisdom in the industry.

For those of us who have experienced medical errors firsthand or loss of a loved one at the hands of an experienced healthcare provider, this is especially difficult. However, without this mindset the victim mentality can quickly take over and all pro-active efforts are futile. It would be remiss not to acknowledge that every healthcare professional or provider is in love with their profession and yes, there are some providers that are better than others, as with any profession.

With this critical perspective in mind, we start Step Two with the vision and mindset that the majority of professionals are exactly that – professionals with a mission to help and heal.

Step Two: Determine if you or a loved one need help

If you have a cold or a cough, (non-COVID related) determining the next steps to feel better is often a well-known path of action. Over the counter options, telehealth and other remedies often come into mind. Vitamin C, and other natural remedies are often employed to try and combat the common cold. However, a more complicated scenario like COVID, or multiple health issues and/or a chronic illness, will require research, the input and opinions of qualified individuals along with access to the best care. This can become overwhelming and frustrating, quickly. This is where you may want to consider becoming a navigator/advocate or engaging one if:

- You don't fully understand the problem, illness or situation and multiple providers are involved

- You have critical decisions to make and your providers aren't sharing the level of information you need

- You're emotionally involved and unable to clearly see facts vs. a loved one or your own healthcare situation in a fair light

- The diagnosis is progressive such as cancer, Alzheimer's, Parkinson's or other chronic disease that has a path of progression

- You have responsibilities that will prevent you from investing the amount of time necessary to effectively handle the situation at hand

- The insurance company isn't able to explain the plan, benefits and options in a way that is understandable for you

These are all scenarios where you could consider engaging a navigator or advocate to help you navigate these unchartered waters with more clarity and peace of mind.

Step Three: Become an advocate or obtain one

Become your own healthcare advocate/navigator or obtain one from an organization who specializes in this. Advocates can be:

- YOU! Take classes or use your experience and the resources offered in The Prepared Patient Prescription™ and the justforpatients. org site to serve as your own advocate or for your loved one. Take time to educate yourself on how to best advocate in your situation and insure you have the time and resources to devote to it. If not, move on to the next option, which is to hire one.

- Seek out a qualified navigator/advocate from an organization that provides this service either as a non-profit at no cost, or for hire. These individuals are qualified and possibly certified with experience. Often, they are nursing professionals and/or doctors who have retired after many years in the healthcare field. Educated, knowledgeable and eager to help but unable to serve in the demanding capacity the healthcare industry often requires. But they make amazing navigators and advocates. Why? They know the system, the resources and tools available to you. They understand the vernacular and processes needed to be successful. They have experience. Enlist a friend or relative with a level of experience that will suffice based on the situation and the motivation to invest the time and resources to research/facilitate on your behalf. This is someone who can serve with an objective, neutral position and has some working knowledge of the healthcare systems. In order for this to work, both you/patient and the friend/relative will set ground rules and boundaries for engagement and interaction, as well as when it would be ok to act on behalf of the patient. In these cases, a medical power of attorney may be utilized, but not always.

As a rule of thumb, navigators and advocates should:

- ✓ Act appropriately in medical situations on your behalf

- ✓ Equipped to ask relevant questions

- ✓ Follow through to ensure the answers are appropriate

- ✓ Provide information to help make a decision

- ✓ Be an active listener; willing to learn, help and be open to new ideas

- ✓ Be an assertive communicator

- ✓ Have the ability to employ critical thinking quickly

- ✓ Be able to coordinate activities on multiple levels with a sense of peace, purpose and intention

- ✓ Optimally, a navigator/advocate would be someone with a healthcare background who understand the systems, procedures, process and reporting

- ✓ Ability to provide emotional support during a routine office visit or medical emergency

Step Four: Capture Your Medical Journey and History

Create a medical journal for yourself and your loved ones. The Prepared Patient Journal™ or app is an inexpensive way to journal and capture every visit, incident, accident, discussion, injury, surgery or routine exam in one place. This is also the place to record medications, allergies and other supplements taken now or in the past.

Whether you have one doctor or several, a physical book or an app, this journal will be your "medical history single point of contact" that will accompany you to any doctor or healthcare provider visit or telehealth appointment. It captures what tests have been done recently, immunizations, prescriptions, supplements and more. It serves as a holistic view of you or the patient's healthcare landscape.

Something that is almost but not fully 100% in place are Electronic Health Records, which were required by law in 2015. "An electronic health record (EHR) is a digital version of a patient's paper chart. EHRs are real-time, patient-centered records that make information available instantly and securely to authorized users. While an EHR does contain the medical and treatment histories of patients, an EHR system is built to go beyond standard clinical data collected in a provider's office and can be inclusive of a broader view of a patient's care. EHRs are a vital part of health IT and can contain a patient's medical history, diagnoses, medications, treatment plans, immunization dates, allergies, radiology images, and laboratory and test results. It can also allow access to evidence-based tools that providers can use to make decisions about a patient's care. In addition, it automates and streamlines provider workflow.[19]

"As recently as 2012, an estimated 63% of physicians were still using the fax machine as a primary means of communication, a statistic that may be mind-boggling to those outside the health care industry. But in today's digital age, with more and more doctors using electronic health records (EHRs), this office dinosaur is finally headed toward extinction—right? Well, maybe. Despite massive effort and investment in health information systems and technology, and many years of widespread availability, the full promised benefits of EHRs are far from fruition. And the reality is that most physicians still have to fax, and mail patient records the way they did a decade ago."[20]

One of the key features of an EHR is that health information can be created and managed by authorized providers in a digital format capable of being shared with other providers across more than one health care organization. EHRs are built to share information with other health care providers and organizations – such as laboratories, specialists, medical imaging facilities, pharmacies, emergency facilities, and school and workplace clinics – so they contain information from all clinicians involved in a patient's care. Hypothetically, using EHR a healthcare professional would have the ability to quickly view allergies, medications, medical conditions, current medical reports like blood tests, CAT scans, emergency contacts, personal doctors and past surgeries, anywhere that took place. In addition, blood type, photo id and .pdf files of any healthcare power of attorney and/or living will could be accessed in case of emergency. Once fully implemented across all healthcare options, EHR could provide on-line access to health records for your medical providers. "As of 2017, nearly 9 in 10 (86%) of office-based physicians had adopted any EHR, and nearly 4 in 5 (80%) had adopted a certified EHR."[21]

97 percent of hospitals nationwide used EHR data in 2017, compared to 87 percent in 2015[22]

EHR does not cancel the responsibility you have to maintain your own records for your own investment in your healthcare options, outcomes and decisions. Ultimately, technology may or may not be relied upon in an emergency situation and your knowledge and personal journals will be of utmost value.

The Prepared Patient Prescription™

Step **One** – Acknowledge healthcare professionals
are in the business to help

Step **Two** – Determine if you or a loved one need help

Step **Three** – Become an advocate or obtain one

Step **Four** – Capture Your Medical Journey and History

CHAPTER 4

Talking with Your Healthcare Professional and Getting the Answers You Need

ROSEMARY'S STORY

...A few days before her passing, Rosemary was on the road to recovery. She had rebounded from numerous errors, issues and situations and appeared hopeful about a possible lung transplant to eradicate the effects of COPD as well as getting the hospital, the place she had come to know as home over the past many week. On a routine visit to help with atrophied muscles, well-meaning physical therapists came by to help her regain strength in her legs, arms and other muscles. During this session, they were unaware of the numerous tubes that were placed in her body to compensate for her lack of ability to walk and move about. In the process of therapy, one tube was pushed, and we would later learn, accidentally

ruptured her colon, releasing bacteria and poison into her bloodstream. Later in the day, with a bloodstained bed, she was rushed to an ICU unit. The nurse on duty was unaware of the physical therapy and the ICU staff was also unaware of the therapy, thereby leaving a gap in the cause or the treatment that could have saved her life as sepsis set in.

Talking to a doctor, nurse or other healthcare professional can, at times, be extremely intimidating and confusing. With seven minutes or less to explain concerns, ailments and prior history or medications taken, it's a challenge to ensure you're able to share all the critical information necessary before a diagnosis and potentially a prescription is handed to you.

Feelings of intimidation, insecurity and fear can all cloud the discussions we have with our healthcare professionals. If there is a cultural background difference, language barriers can be present as well. Medical vernacular the professional uses instead of lay terminology may send you sideways and unable to concentrate if you aren't able to clarify what was really said. All of these add up to an experience that does not necessarily end up positively for you as the patient. Unless you or the patient are vocal, a healthcare professional may not know what questions, concerns you have and/or the full history and how it might impact your treatment and diagnosis.

For example, most recently, my family learned we have a pre-disposed gene mutation. Affectionately called the MTHFR mutation, this genetic disposition interferes with absorption of vitamins and minerals. In addition, certain types of anesthesia interact or become ineffective, making surgery a dangerous proposition for someone with this mutation.

One vitamin in particular, Folic Acid, can become poisonous in the body in some cases. Women with this mutation run significant risks when pregnant. "During pregnancy, women who test positive for a mutated MTHFR gene may have a higher risk for miscarriages, preeclampsia, or a baby born with birth defects, such as spina bifida."[23] Keeping 23&Me© information, data and reports in your medical journal and bringing them electronically or hard copy to a healthcare appointment is important and in some cases could be lifesaving.

If you have more than one healthcare provider who are assigned to you or that you have engaged, all have an opportunity to communicate and collaborate to provide holistic healthcare resolutions. When this holistic approach isn't adopted, drug/supplement interactions, missed diagnosis and repeated tests can increase the margin for a medical error or misdiagnosis.

Consider this scenario: My father, while mostly healthy and strong, had a myriad of heart issues and a hip replacement 5 years ago. Bypass surgery, stints and continuous heart medications became his life after those challenges. At times, he takes medication for the pain that remains in his hip after the replacement. He now sees several different healthcare professionals to include a heart doctor, an internal medicine physician, a pain management clinic and an allergist to deal with seasonal allergies.

Recently, my father had been having issues with his prostate and makes an appointment with Dr. J, his internal medicine doctor who prescribed a prostate medication to help. My father didn't have anyone with him at the appointment, or a medical history journal, but this was a routine visit and the prostate issue was not life threatening. He began taking the medication prescribed to alleviate the prostate symptoms and over the course of the next 2 weeks begins fainting, feeling very dizzy most of the time, had trouble focusing his eyesight and experienced several falls as a result. He knew something wasn't right but thought he might have the flu. He stayed inside but did not get better.

In fact, things got worse. He fell and sustained a cut on his left arm. Again, not life threatening, but because he's on blood thinners from his heart doctor, it was difficult to stop the bleeding and took several days of a slow bleed for it to finally clot and stop. Because I'm wasn't convinced, he had the flu given there wasn't a fever, nausea or other common symptoms of the flu, I realized the only thing that changed in his daily regime was the new prostate medication. Concerned, I search the internet about the possibility of the symptoms as a side effect of the medication. Results turned up negative. Curious, I decide to check drug interactions, although I'm certain the doctor, nurse or at least the pharmacist would have checked that before allowing him to take something that might interfere or interact with his other medications. Alarmed, I found the following when asking the internet if blood thinners interact negatively with the prostate medication prescribed:

"may cause fainting, resulting in possible bodily injury and harm"

"nausea"

"dizziness upon standing due to a sudden drop in blood pressure"

"be careful if you drive or do anything that requires you to be alert"

"Avoid standing for long periods of time or becoming overheated during exercise and in hot weather"

"Avoid getting up too fast from a sitting or lying position, or you may feel dizzy"

Whose responsibility was it to ask if these medications interact with each other? The doctor, nurse, pharmacist, your father? All of the above. Back in the early part of this book we outlined that responsibility for your healthcare equally resides with you and the healthcare professionals treating you.

Given what I think I may have learned about the possible interaction, I immediately called the internal medicine doctor's office to let them know what was happening and they agree it's an interaction and prescribe a different drug based on the information I provide related to all the medications my father was taking. The nurse on the phone said, "why didn't your father tell us he was taking other medications?" I agreed and then politely said, "why didn't anyone ask him what medications he was taking before handing out a prescription?" Because...what if **your** father had been driving and passed out and killed others when his car crashed? What if he had been next to the pool or in a bathtub? This could have been a preventable death due to medication interaction, but not easily recognized as such.

What follows next is a tool that will help you get the most out of your telehealth or in person appointments and a way to develop mutually respectful relationships with healthcare providers. This also provides a path to create a holistic view of your healthcare situation, a priority when you need to engage all necessary healthcare providers.

Recommendations for a successful healthcare appointment (in person or telehealth)

1. When booking an appointment, ensure it's clear, concise and understandable. If you have numerous issues to talk about with your physician or provider, let the scheduler know at booking so that an ample amount of time is scheduled for you.

2. Take time to prepare before you attend your appointment. An outline of current issues to discuss, medications and any supplements you are taking is a great starting point. If you are keeping a medical journal, ensure it's up to date with any recent bloodwork, supplements or new exercise regimes. If you are seeing other medical professionals, be sure to have all of that information available as well. Anything you want to make certain you talk to the doctor about, write down and prioritize what's most important. It will be much easier to confirm all your questions and concerns are addressed if you have them in written form.

3. For the topics you'd like to discuss, try to be specific, to the point and fact based in your description of the issues you would like addressed by the healthcare professional. We know that appointments on average are 7 minutes long – by having all your facts, documents and questions clearly outlined and succinct, it will help the healthcare professional reach a more concise conclusion, diagnosis and recommendation. Offer details about significant issues, without being asked. Remember, this is **your** health **or** the health of a loved one.

4. Take time to think and research anything critical prior to your appointment. By doing this research in advance, you'll have the ability to ask relevant questions and to participate in the conversation at a much different level then if you had walked in without any knowledge. While the internet is not always 100% credible, it is a source that can be helpful as well as your local library.

5. Ask the doctor for any written materials or other resources that could be recommended for you to get a better understanding of your diagnosis or next steps. You'll feel more confident and have the ability to be a better advocate for yourself or a loved one.

6. After the appointment, armed with a prescription and/or next steps, write down anything that helps your situation, things that makes it worse or better. If you find that your situation is not improving after the recommended wait time, call and share this information. Depending on the situation, the recommendation may be to schedule another appointment and utilize the same recommendations above for the second visit.

7. There may be times where you feel that your concerns have not been adequately addressed. In this case, reviewing the details of your situation may be helpful to bring clarity and focus on your concerns. If you disagree with the treatment plan or diagnosis, take a moment to clearly outline why. For example, if you are

pregnant and prescribed Folic Acid and you have testing that shows you carry the MTHFR gene mutation, this would be a good time to share this information, if you haven't already. The doctor or other healthcare provider may offer a response which will require you to listen carefully and to take notes. This may change your view. However, if you still continue to feel the treatment plan is not appropriate, it is reasonable to seek another opinion. Most health professionals will welcome this and can be instrumental in facilitating a referral.

With some advance preparation and research as well as confidence that you are empowered to be more in control of the healthcare you receive, you can have a more effective discussion with your healthcare provider. This doesn't require you to possess an aggressive or confrontational personality. By providing facts, offering clarity around details, participating in treatment decisions and following the action plans, you are well on your way to establishing a mutually rewarding and respectful relationship with your doctor and other healthcare professionals.

CHAPTER 5

Becoming A Navigator or Advocate for Yourself or Others

ROSEMARY'S STORY

... As the newest doctor finishes his examination, he says "...she's losing blood but I'm not sure why or where. I think we should put a port in her neck as the one in her arm isn't working well..." Gently and without provocation I ask, "How do the port and the loss of blood correlate?" He responds by shaking his head and saying, "I don't know but if we don't put in the damn port, there will be hell to pay from the nurses..." After the procedure is complete, I walk swiftly to again re-engage the doctor before he enters an elevator. "Was the port insertion successful and what are our next steps?" He stops for a brief moment and glances my way realizing that this daughter isn't giving up for a moment. "The port was successful, and she didn't feel

a thing. As for next steps, let's see how we progress over the next 24 hours." I never saw him again.

The next day, her disposition had worsened. I ask the doctor on call early that morning what is wrong with her? He doesn't know but he does say, "She doesn't have pneumonia. Her lungs are clear and working at typical capacity for her COPD. I've ordered more tests. Let's see what the next 24 hours bring. She may have had a stroke; I don't know yet." ....3 hours later, a doctor pulls me outside the room and says she's already passed. Her heart is just beating with the electricity still in her body. If we disconnect the machines, she will pass quickly. I must make an informed decision. How do I do that? So many confusing and disconnected conversations over the past 24 hours about her stability, what was wrong or not wrong, what the plan of action would or could be. Nothing was making sense. And now... she had passed? Why and how did this happen? Was anyone talking to each other? Were they assessing her condition, charts and if so, why do they not know what had transpired?

Step 1: Education

One of the first steps to becoming an advocate for yourself or a loved one involves education. Understanding in general what to expect from the time you jump on a telehealth call, enter a doctor's office, urgent care or a hospital thru the end of the appointment or discharge, is one key to an optimal healthcare experience.

In some instances, healthcare providers have this information available and clearly outline expectations and/or how to obtain additional information. But with budget cuts that frequently happen, the process of patient education falls short of meeting the needs in some cases.

Knowing what to expect during a telehealth call, a doctor's office or in advance of a hospital visit/ procedure can help to reduce the normal anxiety that accompanies these activities. It also helps you to clearly outline what your concerns are ahead of time and ensure your questions get answered. It can be a benefit to both the healthcare provider and you/your loved one.

Note: As of this printing, COVID is raging throughout the world. The only people allowed in a hospital room or ER is the patient. Advocating for yourself or loved one in this situation is notably more difficult and requires an almost superhuman level of patience and persistence. Using a hired volunteer or paid advocate is increasingly important in this environment because they can help you make a remote plan, outline a clarifying conversation with a healthcare provider that will take place via video or phone, potentially asking all the right questions as well as advice on how best to navigate the situation remotely. If you are the patient, many hospitals have advocates and navigators on staff that may be available to assist you.

Step 2: Creating a Healthcare Support Team

A healthcare support team are not only the healthcare professionals that provide your care but others including you, your involved family members and/or an advocate that you may enlist to help you navigate the healthcare system.

If it's not possible to enlist others support, it is critical to remember that YOU are the most important part of your healthcare team! This is your body, your medical issues and you should feel empowered to ask questions, gain clarity where discussions are not clear and provide input to your care. Partnering with your doctors and nurses will help to keep the lines of communication open and a provide more peaceful experience during times that could have otherwise been stressful due to lack of information or an understanding of the plan for your health.

As noted in the previous chapter, some hospitals and doctor's offices provide patient liaisons or even advocates. Asking an administrator or front desk staff member will most often get you connected with the right department or person to join your healthcare support team.

Step 3: Expectations and Preparations for A Healthcare Provider Visit ~ For The Patient's Use or An Advocate

By investing planning time prior to a doctor visit via telehealth or in person, you increase the odds that that your questions will be answered and you're ready to fully listen to the recommendations for you. In doing so, you also let the doctor know that you are engaged and an active part of your healthcare team. You strengthen your partnership as a participating member of the team.

Using your medical journal, document your questions and/or any changes since your last discussion/visit. You can also clearly outline the reason for the call/visit and what you hope to resolve. I've included a sample in the Appendix, or you can utilize, "The Prepared Patient Medical Journal" to plan for this engagement. This journal also tracks medications so that if a new medication is prescribed you can discuss with your doctor any potential drug interactions.

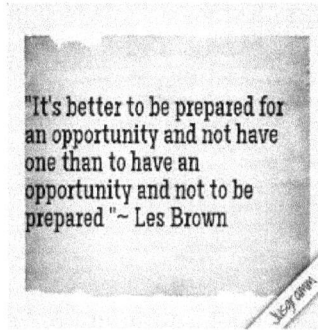

"It's better to be prepared for an opportunity and not have one than to have an opportunity and not to be prepared "~ Les Brown

Step 4: Prior to and during a doctor's call or visit what you can potentially expect as a patient

Considerations as you prepare and attend a healthcare providers office, under normal circumstances (non-pandemic). These are in general and not in any way construed to be an absolute. They are provided as a way to prepare and set an expectation in advance.

- You should be seen in a timely manner when you're sick. This seems like an obvious expectation when you call your healthcare provider, but statistics show it doesn't always happen this way. If you call the doctor's office saying you're not well, you should expect a phone call back from a doctor or nurse within

24 hours. It does not always happen this way, but it is a reasonable expectation according to the National Patient Safety Foundation.

- Your doctor should explain everything in terms you can understand and if not, be prepared with confidence or an advocate who can ask for clarity. "Patients should have a basic expectation that they're going to be provided information they need in terms they understand," says Diane Pinakiewicz, president of the National Patient Safety Foundation.[24]

- Every procedure that is done to your body or handled on your behalf should be preceded with an explanation as to what it is under evaluation and how it will be done. The experts we talked to say your healthcare provider should clearly state what's going to happen, the medication you'll be receiving and any significant side effects, even ones that aren't dangerous, but could be annoying, like a dry mouth.

If it's not: Your job is to ask questions prior to any procedure or medication being prescribed.

Questions to ask prior to any procedure, test or surgery:

- Can you explain what the procedure is you're about to do and how it will be done

- What do you hope to determine from this procedure

- What can I expect in terms of pain or possible side effects

  - If severe effects, another question would be:

    - Is this the only procedure that will get the answers you are seeking

    - Is this absolutely necessary

    - Are there any alternatives to this procedure that may has less side effects, less pain or minimally invasive?

- You should expect your results within a timely manner.

According to the National Patient Safety foundation[25], you should hear test results within 48 hours of when the results come into your doctor's office or sooner if it's an urgent issue. Simple lab work is often done in a day. More complicated tests can take a week or longer.

- *Your job is to ask when the results will be back.*

- It's reasonable to expect the doctor to call you with the results, especially if they are not positive in nature. Most in the industry feel the doctor should call you even if the results are positive, given the test results can lead to changes in your overall treatment plans.

- Every medication that is prescribed or administered should be named, and a clear explanation of what the medication will do, along with potential side effects – in advance. Printed prescription education material should accompany any prescription prescribed or administered.

- If there is a change in your condition either at

the doctor's office or a facility and a new plan of care is created, you and your healthcare support team should have input into it.

- Remember: Your medical professionals are also your teachers.

APPENDIX

Resources to help you or a loved one advocate for
healthcare situations

Healthcare Journal Pages

The following is a sample of the type of information you can expect to collect as part of your Medical History Journal. Document this information for your use at a regular healthcare visit, Urgent Care or Emergency Room.

Purpose of the Visit
Setting (office, ER, hospital)
What issue(s) are you being seen for
What makes the issue worse or better
What medications have you taken either over

the counter or prescribed
How does the current issue(s) affect your life?
What could you do before that you can't do

now (unable to work, unable to walk, loss of

appetite, etc.)
Associated symptoms
Any other symptoms occurring since the

current illness started

What was happening before this issue began

(new medication, new exercise program, family

challenges, work issues)
In your opinion what do you think the issue

could be

Becoming Your Own Navigator or Advocate <u>or</u> Advocating for A Loved One

Before you take on the navigator or advocate role, here are questions to consider:

In an emergency or a regular doctor's office telehealth conversation or in person visit do you feel empowered to ask questions?

If so and the answer is confusing or not in laymen's terms do you feel empowered to let the doctor know you didn't understand and need him/her to explain in a different style?

Do you write out the answers and track the recommended course of action from that visit or healthcare situation?

Do you feel empowered to get a second opinion, if only thru a phone call to another healthcare provider?

If you answered no to any of these questions you may want to consider enlisting a professionally trained advocate or competent loved one to attend office visits and/or be available in case of an emergency.

Routine Healthcare Follow-up Telehealth Call or Visit Template
Are you having any symptoms that suggest that your problem is getting worse?
List your current medicines (name, dosage, and number of times taken per day).
Describe any problems you have had in taking your medicines as prescribed.
Are you having any undesirable side effects from your medicines?

Record any relevant measurements such as blood sugar or blood pressure readings. A spreadsheet or table showing the trends in these measurements over time can be helpful to your physician (See the sample spreadsheet on last page).

Questions to consider asking:

How Do I Get My Results of Tests ...

Does My Family History Put Me At Risk? ...

Am I Old/Young enough For That? ...

Is Stress Impacting My Health? If so, what
resources are available to me to mitigate? ...

How Is My Weight? ...

What Vaccinations Do I Need? ...

Are My Habits Harmful? Are there habits that need
to stop or start?...

Are My Prescriptions Still Relevant or Interacting?

The following isn't meant to be completed in this book but represents information to capture for you or a loved one. You can capture this info in a notebook or the workbook on www.justforpatients.org

Medical History Information Collection Template		
First Illness or Injury:		
Date:	Treating physician:	
How treated:		
Second Illness or Significant injury:		
Date:	Treating physician:	
How treated:		
Third Illness or Significant injury:		
Date:	Treating physician:	
How treated:		
Other hospitalizations		
Reason for first hospitalization:		
Dates:	Hospital:	
Reason for second hospitalization:		
Dates:	Hospital:	
Reason for third hospitalization:		
Dates:	Hospital:	
Do you have any history of?		
Heart diseaseYes No	Date started:	How treated:
Diabetes Yes No	Date started:	How treated:

CancerYes No	Date stared:	How treated:
COPD Yes No	Date Started:	How Treated:
COVID Yes No	Date Started:	How Treated:

Do you have any allergies?¨ Yes ¨ No If yes, please list them below.	
Cause:	Type of reaction:
Cause:	Type of reaction:
Cause:	Type of reaction:

Are there any medications you cannot take?¨ Yes ¨ No If yes, please list them below.	
Medication:	Type of reaction:
Medication:	Type of reaction:
Medication:	Type of reaction:

Current prescription medications		
Name:	Dosage (mg):	Times per day:
Name:	Dosage (mg):	Times per day:
Name:	Dosage (mg):	Times per day:

Current over-the-counter medications		
Name:	Dosage (mg):	Times per day:
Name:	Dosage (mg):	Times per day:

Name:	Dosage (mg):	Times per day:
Current vitamins, supplements, or herbal products		
Name:	Dosage (mg):	Times per day:
Name:	Dosage (mg):	Times per day:
Name:	Dosage (mg):	Times per day:
Immunizations		
Date of last Tetanus/ Diphtheria vaccination:		
Date of last Pneumonia vaccination:		
Date of last flu shot:		
Family Medical History		
Mother	Current age:	
Significant illnesses:		
If deceased age at death:	Cause of death:	
Father	Current Age:	
Significant illnesses:		
If deceased age at death:	Cause of death:	
Sibling 1: ¨ brother ¨ sister	Current Age:	
Significant illnesses:		
If deceased, age at death:	Cause of death:	

Notes for Healthcare Providers

Enlisting the assistance of a Patient Navigator or Patient Advocate

www.justforpatients.org where you can find access to resources, content and people who can help.

References

1   https://www.cnbc.com/2018/02/22/medical-errors-third-leading-cause-of-death-in-america.html
2   https://www.cnbc.com/2018/02/22/medical-errors-third-leading-cause-of-death-in-america.html
3   https://money.cnn.com/2018/05/04/news/economy/health-care-workers-shortage/index.html
4   https://money.cnn.com/2018/05/04/news/economy/health-care-workers-shortage/index.html
5   https://online.regiscollege.edu/blog/importance-communication-health-care/
6   https://online.regiscollege.edu/blog/importance-communication-health-care/
7   https://www.audible.com/author/Edward-T-Creagan/B001IR1LE8
8   https://www.mercatus.org/publications/healthcare/affordable-care-act-2014-significant-insurer-losses-despite-substantial
9   Seema Verma, administrator of the Centers for Medicare and Medicaid Services, Washington, Sept. 27, 2018
10 https://www.npr.org/sections/health-shots/2019/10/14/768731628/trump-is-trying-hard-to-thwart-obamacare-hows-that-going
11 https://www.npr.org/sections/health-shots/2019/10/14/768731628/trump-is-trying-hard-to-thwart-obamacare-hows-that-going
12 https://thepapergown.zocdoc.com/the-biggest-healthcare-changes-under-trump/
14 https://thepapergown.zocdoc.com/the-biggest-healthcare-changes-under-trump/
15 https://thepapergown.zocdoc.com/the-biggest-healthcare-changes-under-trump/
16 https://www.healthmarkets.com/resources/health-insurance/trumpcare-news-updates/

17 https://www.parents.com/parenting/money/insurance/tips-to-get-the-most-out-of-your-health-insurance/

18 https://www.parents.com/parenting/money/insurance/tips-to-get-the-most-out-of-your-health-insurance/

19 https://www.healthit.gov/faq/what-electronic-health-record-ehr

20 https://www.ncbi.nlm.nih.gov/pmc/articles/PMC5565131/

21 https://dashboard.healthit.gov/quickstats/quickstats.php

22 https://ehrintelligence.com/news/most-hospitals-use-ehr-data-to-support-quality-improvement-efforts

23 https://www.healthline.com/health/pregnancy/mth-fr#about-mthfr

24 http://www.ihi.org/about/news/Pages/npsf-and-ihi-to-merge-in-may.aspx

25 http://www.ihi.org/about/news/Pages/npsf-and-ihi-to-merge-in-may.aspx

www.ingramcontent.com/pod-product-compliance
Lightning Source LLC
Chambersburg PA
CBHW072154020426
42334CB00018B/2006